I0707007

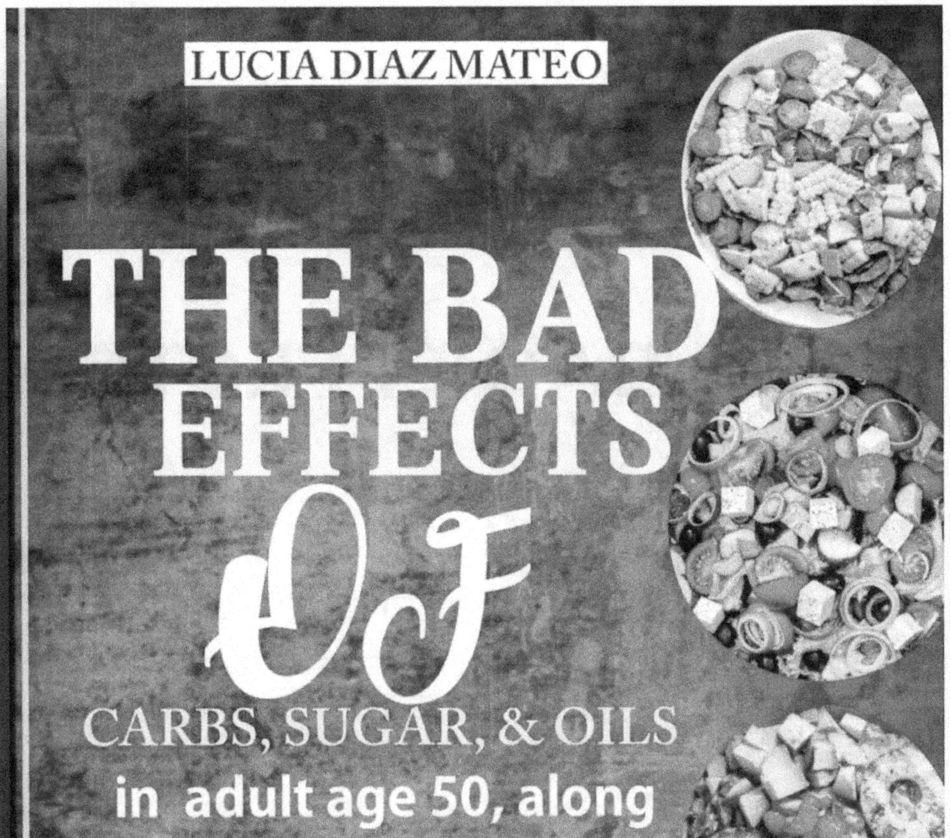
LUCIA DIAZ MATEO
THE BAD
EFFECTS
OF
CARBS, SUGAR, & OILS
in adult age 50, along with sugar-free diabetic treats for adults, and how to escape their control

THE BAD EFFECTS

of **Carbs, Sugar, And Oils** In Adult **Age 50**, along with sugar-free **diabetic** treats for adults, and how to escape their control

LUCIA DIAZ MATEO

Copyright ©

All rights reserved.

No part of this publication may be reproduced, distributed, or transmitted in any form or by any means, including photocopying, recording, or other electronic or mechanical methods, without the prior written permission of the publisher, except as permitted by U.S. copyright law. For permission requests, contact the author For privacy reasons,some names, locations, and dates may have been changed.

CONTENTS

CHAPTER 1. INTRODUCTION

The introduction serves as the gateway to our exploration of the detrimental effects of carbohydrates, sugar, and oils on adults at the age of 50, particularly those dealing with diabetes.

In today's fast-paced world, where dietary choices are abundant and often convenience-driven, understanding the impact of these components on the health of individuals aged 50 and above is of paramount importance. This section will delve into the overarching purpose of our analysis and underscore why addressing the influence of carbs, sugar, and oils is crucial for the well-being of this specific demographic.

1.1 Overview of the Analysis

Our analysis aims to dissect the intricate relationship between dietary choices and the health outcomes of adults reaching the age of 50, a phase where metabolic changes and susceptibility to certain health issues become more prominent. By examining the science behind carbohydrates, sugar, and oils, we intend to shed light on the mechanisms that contribute to negative health effects and how they may impact individuals differently as they age.

1.2 Importance of Addressing the Impact

Understanding the significance of addressing the impact of carbs, sugar, and oils on adults at age 50 is pivotal for public health initiatives and individual well-being. The introduction will emphasize the broader implications of unhealthy dietary habits, setting the stage for a comprehensive exploration of each component's consequences. By acknowledging the importance of this analysis, readers will gain insight into why these dietary factors need careful consideration, especially in the context of the aging population.

This section will also touch upon the prevalence of diabetes in adults over 50, highlighting the increased vulnerability of this demographic to metabolic challenges. By framing the discussion within the context of diabetes, we draw attention to the specific health concerns that amplify the importance of making informed dietary choices.

In essence, the introduction serves as a call to action, urging readers to recognize the significance of our exploration and its potential impact on individual health and societal well-being. It sets the tone for an in-depth examination of how carbs, sugar, and oils influence the health trajectory of adults at age 50 and establishes the foundation for the subsequent chapters that will delve into each component's effects in detail.

Chapter 2: Carbohydrates and Blood Sugar Levels

2.1 High Carbohydrate Intake: A Double-Edged Sword

Carbohydrates are a fundamental component of our diet, providing the body with essential energy. However, for adults aged 50 and above, the impact of high carbohydrate intake becomes a critical concern. As we age, our metabolism tends to slow down, making it crucial to monitor the quantity and quality of carbohydrates consumed.

Excessive carbohydrate intake can lead to a surge in blood sugar levels, posing a significant risk for individuals in this age group. While carbohydrates are essential for energy, the body's ability to process them diminishes over time. This can result in an imbalance between energy intake and expenditure, contributing to weight gain and potential complications, especially for those with diabetes.

Moreover, the type of carbohydrates consumed plays a crucial role. Refined carbohydrates, such as those found in sugary snacks and processed foods, can cause rapid spikes in blood sugar levels. This, in turn, puts additional stress on the body's insulin response, potentially leading to insulin resistance—a precursor to diabetes.

2.2 Elevated Blood Sugar Levels in Adults at Age 50

For adults aged 50 and above, maintaining stable blood sugar levels is paramount to overall health. Elevated blood sugar levels, known as hyperglycemia, can have various adverse effects on the body. One of the immediate concerns is the impact on cognitive function. Studies have shown a correlation between elevated blood sugar levels and cognitive decline in older adults, emphasizing the importance of managing carbohydrate intake.

Furthermore, persistent hyperglycemia can lead to complications such as cardiovascular issues and damage to blood vessels, increasing the risk of heart disease. For individuals with diabetes, the challenge is even more pronounced, as the body's ability to regulate blood sugar is compromised.

Addressing these concerns involves adopting a balanced approach to carbohydrate consumption. Choosing complex carbohydrates with a lower glycemic index, such as whole grains, legumes, and vegetables, can provide sustained energy without causing drastic spikes in blood sugar levels. This nuanced approach to carbohydrate intake is especially relevant for adults at age 50 and beyond, contributing to better overall health and diabetes management.

Chapter 3: Carbs and Insulin Resistance

Carbohydrates play a crucial role in providing energy for the body, but the relationship between carbs and insulin resistance becomes particularly significant for adults at age 50 and above.

3.1 Link Between High Glycemic Index Carbs:

Carbohydrates are classified based on their glycemic index (GI), a measure of how quickly they raise blood sugar levels. High glycemic index carbs, such as refined grains and sugary foods, can lead to rapid spikes in blood sugar. In individuals aged 50 and above, these spikes can pose a considerable risk, contributing to insulin resistance.

The body's ability to regulate blood sugar diminishes with age, making older adults more susceptible to the negative effects of high GI carbs. When consumed regularly, these carbs can overwhelm the insulin response, leading to insulin resistance—a condition where the cells no longer respond efficiently to insulin, resulting in elevated blood sugar levels.

3.2 Insulin Resistance in Older Adults:

Insulin resistance is a common concern for adults over 50, and its relationship with carbohydrates is multifaceted. As the body ages, cells become less responsive to insulin's signaling, making it challenging to regulate glucose effectively. High carbohydrate intake exacerbates this issue, creating a cycle of insulin resistance that can contribute to the development of type 2 diabetes.

Moreover, insulin resistance is associated with increased inflammation, a phenomenon that becomes more prevalent with age. Chronic inflammation is linked to various health problems, including cardiovascular issues and metabolic disorders. Understanding this intricate interplay between high glycemic index carbs and insulin resistance is crucial for developing effective strategies to mitigate these risks in older adults.

Strategies to Mitigate Carbs-Induced Insulin Resistance in Older Adults:

1. Emphasizing Low-Glycemic Carbs: Encouraging the consumption of low-glycemic index carbohydrates, such as whole grains, legumes, and non-starchy vegetables, can help regulate blood sugar levels more effectively in older adults.

2. Portion Control: Managing portion sizes is crucial for preventing excessive carb intake. Smaller, balanced meals spread throughout the day can promote steady blood sugar levels and reduce the risk of insulin resistance.

3. Incorporating Fiber: Including fiber-rich foods in the diet, such as fruits, vegetables, and whole grains, can slow down the absorption of sugars and improve overall glycemic control.

4. Regular Monitoring and Adjustments: For individuals with diabetes or those at risk of insulin resistance, regular monitoring of blood sugar levels

is essential. Adjustments to the diet and lifestyle can be made based on these readings to maintain optimal glucose levels.

Chapter 4: Detrimental Effects of Sugar

the multifaceted and detrimental effects of sugar consumption, particularly its impact on adults aged 50 and above. Understanding how sugar contributes to obesity, cardiovascular issues, increased insulin resistance, and inflammation is crucial for individuals seeking to manage their health effectively.

4.1 Obesity and Cardiovascular Issues:

Excessive sugar intake has been linked to the rising prevalence of obesity, a health concern that becomes even more pronounced in individuals aged 50 and above. The body's metabolism undergoes changes with age, making it more susceptible to weight gain. High sugar content in the diet contributes to calorie surplus, leading to adipose tissue accumulation.

Furthermore, the relationship between sugar and cardiovascular issues is undeniable. The overconsumption of added sugars is associated with elevated triglyceride levels and a decrease in high-density lipoprotein (HDL) cholesterol, increasing the risk of heart disease. Exploring these connections provides valuable insights into the importance of sugar moderation, especially for older adults concerned about their cardiovascular health.

4.2 Increased Insulin Resistance in Individuals Aged 50 and Above:

Aging itself is a factor that can contribute to insulin resistance, and when coupled with high sugar consumption, the risks are heightened. Insulin resistance, a key component of type 2 diabetes, occurs when cells fail to respond effectively to insulin. For adults at age 50 and above, this phenomenon can exacerbate existing metabolic challenges.

Sugar, particularly in the form of refined carbohydrates, prompts spikes in blood glucose levels, demanding increased insulin production. Over time, the body's insulin response weakens, leading to elevated blood sugar levels and, eventually, insulin resistance. Unraveling this intricate relationship sheds light on the importance of managing sugar intake for older adults, especially those at risk of or living with diabetes.

4.3 Sugar's Role in Inflammation and Chronic Health Conditions During Aging:

Inflammation is a natural response in the body, but chronic inflammation is linked to various health issues, including those associated with aging. Sugar has been identified as a pro-inflammatory substance, contributing to the development and progression of chronic conditions.

In older adults, the aging process itself induces a state of low-grade inflammation. Excessive sugar consumption can exacerbate this inflammation, leading to increased oxidative stress and damage to cells. Understanding how sugar acts as a catalyst for inflammation is essential for individuals seeking to mitigate the risks of chronic health conditions, such as arthritis and cardiovascular diseases, that become more prevalent with age.

Chapter 5: Unhealthy Oils and Cardiovascular Problems

The impact of trans fats and saturated fats on cardiovascular health is of paramount concern, and understanding these dynamics is crucial for individuals seeking to improve their well-being.

5.1 Cardiovascular Problems Associated with Trans Fats:

Trans fats, often found in partially hydrogenated oils, have been extensively linked to cardiovascular issues.

For adults over the age of 50, the risks associated with these fats become more pronounced. Trans fats are notorious for increasing LDL (low-density lipoprotein) cholesterol while simultaneously decreasing HDL (high-density lipoprotein) cholesterol. This imbalance heightens the risk of atherosclerosis, a condition characterized by the buildup of plaque in arteries, potentially leading to heart attacks and strokes.

As individuals age, their cardiovascular system undergoes natural changes, including reduced elasticity of blood vessels and an increased likelihood of hypertension.

The introduction of trans fats exacerbates these age-related changes, posing a significant threat to heart health. The chapter explores the biochemical processes through which trans fats contribute to arterial plaque formation and the subsequent cardiovascular consequences.

5.2 Saturated Fats and Their Impact on Older Adults:

Saturated fats, predominantly found in animal products and certain oils, present another challenge to cardiovascular health, particularly for those aged 50 and above. These fats are known to raise total cholesterol levels, including both LDL and HDL cholesterol. While the impact of saturated fats on cholesterol is well-established, the interplay between aging and these fats requires nuanced consideration.

That's investigates how saturated fats may contribute to the progression of atherosclerosis in older adults and explores potential mechanisms that make this age group more susceptible to the detrimental effects of such fats. Additionally, it addresses the importance of dietary choices in managing saturated fat intake and maintaining heart health in the later stages of life.

Chapter 6: Inflammation Caused by Unhealthy Oils

Inflammation, a complex biological response to harmful stimuli, plays a crucial role in the body's defense mechanism. However, when chronic and uncontrolled, inflammation can lead to various health issues, particularly in adults aged 50 and above.

6.1 The Role of Inflammation in Aging

As the body ages, the immune system undergoes changes that can contribute to a state of chronic inflammation. This process, often referred to as "inflammaging,"

 is associated with a higher prevalence of chronic diseases, including diabetes. Unhealthy dietary habits, especially the consumption of oils rich in trans fats and saturated fats, can exacerbate this inflammatory state.

6.2 Unraveling the Link Between Unhealthy Oils and Inflammation

6.2.1 Trans Fats and Inflammation

Trans fats, commonly found in partially hydrogenated oils, have long been recognized as a major contributor to inflammation.

These artificial fats not only increase levels of inflammatory markers but also decrease those with anti-inflammatory properties.

In older adults, whose bodies may already be predisposed to inflammation, the consumption of trans fats can amplify the inflammatory response.

6.2.2 Saturated Fats and Inflammatory Processes

Saturated fats, prevalent in various cooking oils and animal products, can also play a role in promoting inflammation.

Studies suggest that these fats may trigger inflammatory pathways, leading to increased levels of cytokines and other inflammatory markers.

The aging process intensifies this effect, making older individuals more susceptible to the inflammatory consequences of saturated fat consumption.

6.3 Impact of Unhealthy Oils on Individuals with Diabetes

For adults aged 50 and above, especially those with diabetes, the implications of inflammation caused by unhealthy oils become even more critical.

Diabetes is characterized by chronic inflammation, and consuming oils that exacerbate this condition can heighten the risk of complications.

Inflammation can compromise insulin sensitivity, worsen glycemic control, and contribute to the progression of diabetes-related complications.

6.4 Strategies to Mitigate Inflammation Caused by Unhealthy Oils

Understanding the link between unhealthy oils and inflammation prompts the need for strategies to mitigate these effects.

Incorporating healthier cooking oils, such as olive oil rich in monounsaturated fats, can be a positive step.

Additionally, increasing the intake of omega-3 fatty acids, found in fatty fish like salmon and flaxseeds, has been associated with anti-inflammatory benefits.

6.5 The Importance of Balanced Dietary Choices

Adopting a balanced diet that prioritizes whole foods and minimizes the consumption of processed and fried foods is paramount. The Mediterranean diet, renowned for its anti-inflammatory properties, emphasizes the consumption of fruits, vegetables, nuts, and olive oil.

Integrating these dietary principles can contribute to reducing inflammation and promoting overall health, especially for adults aged 50 and above.

6.6 Collaborative Efforts for Inflammation Management

Managing inflammation caused by unhealthy oils requires a multidisciplinary approach. Healthcare professionals, including physicians and nutritionists, play a pivotal role in providing personalized guidance.

Tailoring dietary recommendations to individual health conditions, considering factors such as diabetes and age, is essential for effective inflammation management.

Chapter 7. Benefits of Zero Sugar Diabetic Snacks

In the realm of managing diabetes, the role of dietary choices is paramount. For individuals aged 50 and above, especially those grappling with diabetes, zero sugar diabetic snacks emerge as a crucial ally in promoting not just enjoyable eating experiences but also in contributing to better health outcomes.

7.1 Advantages of Diabetic Snacks with Zero Sugar

Diabetes, a metabolic disorder characterized by elevated blood sugar levels, necessitates a vigilant approach to dietary selections. Zero sugar diabetic snacks, designed specifically to cater to the needs of individuals with diabetes, offer several distinct advantages.

7.1.1 Blood Sugar Management

The primary benefit of zero sugar diabetic snacks lies in their ability to aid in managing blood sugar levels. By eliminating added sugars, these snacks help prevent sudden spikes in blood glucose, providing a more stable and controlled environment for individuals with diabetes. This is particularly crucial for adults at age 50, where maintaining stable blood sugar levels becomes increasingly challenging.

7.1.2 Weight Management

Weight management is often a critical aspect of diabetes care, and zero sugar snacks contribute significantly to this endeavor. These snacks are typically lower in calories and can be part of a well-balanced diet, supporting weight control efforts for individuals aged 50 and above who are more susceptible to weight-related health issues.

7.1.3 Reduced Risk of Cardiovascular Complications

Diabetes and cardiovascular issues often go hand in hand. Zero sugar diabetic snacks, by avoiding added sugars and unhealthy fats, play a role in reducing the risk of cardiovascular complications. This is of particular importance for adults over 50, as the prevalence of cardiovascular problems tends to increase with age.

7.2 Managing Blood Sugar Levels with Healthier Alternatives

7.2.1 Incorporating Natural Sweeteners

Zero sugar diabetic snacks often utilize natural sweeteners like stevia or monk fruit. These alternatives not only impart sweetness without affecting blood sugar levels but also bring additional health benefits. Stevia, for instance, has been associated with antioxidant and anti-inflammatory properties, offering a potential dual benefit for individuals with diabetes.

7.2.2 High Fiber Content

Fiber plays a pivotal role in glycemic control. Many zero sugar snacks are rich in fiber, contributing to a slower release of glucose into the bloodstream. This slow release helps in avoiding rapid spikes in blood sugar levels, providing a more sustained and regulated energy source.

7.2.3 Nutrient-Dense Options

Beyond just being sugar-free, diabetic snacks often prioritize nutrient density. This means that even though they may lack added sugars, they can still provide essential vitamins, minerals, and other micronutrients. This nutritional profile supports overall health and well-being, addressing the specific nutritional needs of adults at age 50.

7.3 Overcoming Taste Concerns

One common misconception about diabetic snacks, particularly those with zero sugar, is that they may compromise on taste. However, advancements in food science and culinary techniques have led to the development of flavorful and satisfying options that cater to diverse palates.

7.3.1 Culinary Innovations

In recent years, the food industry has seen an influx of culinary innovations in the diabetic snack category. Chefs and food scientists are employing creative approaches to enhance flavors without relying on traditional sugars. This ensures that individuals can enjoy snacks that are not only diabetes-friendly but also delectable.

7.3.2 Diverse Product Offerings

The market for zero sugar diabetic snacks has expanded significantly, providing a diverse array of options. From savory to sweet, crunchy to chewy, individuals have the opportunity to choose snacks that align with their taste preferences. This variety is crucial in ensuring that adherence to a diabetic-friendly diet does not become monotonous or restrictive.

7.4 Incorporating Zero Sugar Snacks into Daily Life

Adopting a lifestyle that includes zero sugar diabetic snacks requires a thoughtful and practical approach. Here are some strategies to seamlessly incorporate these snacks into daily life:

7.4.1 Snack Planning

Planning snacks in advance can help individuals make intentional and healthy choices. Having a variety of zero sugar options readily available ensures that there are always satisfying and diabetes-friendly choices at hand.

7.4.2 Portion Control

While zero sugar snacks offer health benefits, it's essential to practice portion control. Even healthy snacks can contribute to excess calorie intake if consumed in large quantities. Being mindful of portions helps maintain a balanced overall diet.

7.4.3 Balanced Meal Composition

Incorporating zero sugar snacks as part of a balanced diet is key. Combining these snacks with a mix of whole foods, lean proteins, and vegetables ensures a comprehensive nutritional profile, supporting overall health and diabetes management.

Chapter 8: Fiber-Rich and Low-Carb Snack Options

the significance of incorporating fiber-rich and low-carb options into the diet, particularly for adults aged 50 and above, with a focus on managing blood sugar levels and promoting overall well-being.

8.1 Incorporating Fiber-Rich Snacks

The Importance of Fiber:

Fiber plays a crucial role in promoting digestive health, satiety, and blood sugar regulation. For adults at age 50, incorporating fiber-rich snacks can have profound effects on their overall health. Whole grains, fruits, and vegetables are excellent sources of dietary fiber.

Whole Grains as Snack Options:

Opting for whole grain snacks, such as whole wheat crackers or brown rice cakes, provides complex carbohydrates and fiber. These snacks contribute to a slower release of glucose into the bloodstream, helping to maintain stable blood sugar levels.

Fruits and Vegetables:

Snacking on fresh fruits and vegetables not only introduces essential vitamins and minerals but also offers dietary fiber. Examples include apple slices with almond butter or carrot sticks with hummus. These combinations provide a balance of nutrients and help curb unhealthy snack cravings.

8.2 Low-Carb Options for Better Glycemic Control

Understanding Low-Carb Diets:
Low-carb snacks are gaining popularity due to their potential benefits for glycemic control and weight management. For individuals aged 50 and above,

adopting low-carb options can be particularly beneficial in preventing blood sugar spikes.

Nuts and Seeds:

Snacking on nuts and seeds, such as almonds, walnuts, or chia seeds, offers a satisfying crunch along with healthy fats and protein. These snacks are low in carbohydrates and can be a convenient option for those looking to manage their carbohydrate intake.

Recipe: Nutty Crunch Mix

Ingredients:

- 1 cup almonds

- 1 cup walnuts

- 1/2 cup pumpkin seeds

- 1/2 cup sunflower seeds

- 2 tablespoons honey

- 1 tablespoon olive oil

- 1 teaspoon cinnamon

- 1/2 teaspoon sea salt

Instructions:

1. Preheat the Oven:

   Preheat your oven to 325°F (163°C).

2. Prepare the Nuts and Seeds:

In a large mixing bowl, combine the almonds, walnuts, pumpkin seeds, and sunflower seeds. Toss them together to create an even mixture.

3. Create the Sweet and Spicy Coating:

In a small saucepan over low heat, mix honey, olive oil, cinnamon, and sea salt. Stir until the honey is melted and the ingredients are well combined.

4. Coat the Nuts and Seeds:

Pour the honey mixture over the nuts and seeds. Stir well to ensure every piece is coated evenly.

5. Spread on Baking Sheet:

Spread the coated nuts and seeds in a single layer on a baking sheet lined with parchment paper. This ensures they roast evenly.

6. Bake in the Oven:

Place the baking sheet in the preheated oven and bake for 15-20 minutes, or until the nuts and seeds are golden brown. Be sure to stir them every 5 minutes for even roasting.

7. Cool and Break Apart:

Once done, remove the baking sheet from the oven and let the nutty mix cool. As it cools, it will harden and become crunchy. Break it apart into bite-sized clusters.

8. Serve and Enjoy:

Transfer the Nutty Crunch Mix to an airtight container. This delightful snack is ready to be enjoyed at any time. You can serve it on its own or mix it with yogurt, dried fruits, or even sprinkle it on top of salads for an extra crunch.

Tips:

- Experiment with different nuts and seeds based on your preferences.

- Adjust the sweetness and spiciness of the coating by altering the honey and cinnamon quantities.

- Store in an airtight container to maintain freshness.

This Nutty Crunch Mix is not only delicious but also a nutrient-packed snack, providing a satisfying crunch and a combination of healthy fats and protein. Enjoy the benefits of this homemade snack while keeping your blood sugar levels in check.

Greek Yogurt and Berries:

Combining Greek yogurt with berries creates a delicious and low-carb snack. Greek yogurt is rich in protein, which contributes to a feeling of fullness, while berries add natural sweetness and antioxidants without excessive sugar.

Greek Yogurt and Berries Parfait Recipe

Ingredients:

- 1 cup Greek yogurt (unsweetened)

- 1/2 cup mixed berries (strawberries, blueberries, raspberries)

- 1 tablespoon honey (optional, for added sweetness)

- 1/4 cup granola

- Fresh mint leaves for garnish (optional)

Instructions:

1. Prepare the Berries:

   - Wash and slice the strawberries.

   - Rinse the blueberries and raspberries under cold water.

   - Pat the berries dry with a paper towel.

2. Assemble the Parfait:

   - Take a clear glass or a bowl for an aesthetically pleasing presentation.

   - Start by spooning a layer of Greek yogurt into the bottom of the glass.

3. Add a Layer of Berries:

   - Place a few slices of strawberries, a handful of blueberries, and a few raspberries on top of the yogurt layer.

4. Drizzle with Honey (Optional):

- If you prefer a touch of sweetness, drizzle honey over the layer of berries. Adjust the amount based on your taste preferences.

5. Repeat the Layers:

   - Add another layer of Greek yogurt on top of the berries.

   - Follow with another layer of mixed berries.

6. Top with Granola:

   - Sprinkle granola evenly over the berries. This adds a delightful crunch to the parfait and complements the creamy texture of the yogurt.

7. Garnish with Mint Leaves (Optional):

   - For a fresh and visually appealing touch, garnish the top with a few fresh mint leaves.

8. Serve and Enjoy:

   - Your Greek Yogurt and Berries Parfait is now ready to be enjoyed! Serve immediately and savor the delicious combination of creamy yogurt, sweet berries, and crunchy granola.

Tips:

- Use plain Greek yogurt to control added sugars. If you prefer a sweeter taste, opt for honey or a drizzle of maple syrup.

- Experiment with different types of berries or add a mix of nuts for extra flavor and texture.

- Make it a personalized experience by layering the parfait in individual serving glasses for a stylish presentation.

This simple and nutritious Greek Yogurt and Berries Parfait is not only a delightful treat for your taste buds but also a healthy snack option. Enjoy it for breakfast, as a refreshing dessert, or as a midday pick-me-up, knowing that you are indulging in a wholesome and satisfying treat.

Avocado-Based Snacks:

Avocado is a nutrient-dense fruit that is low in carbs and high in healthy fats. Sliced avocado on whole grain toast or as a base for a vegetable dip provides a satisfying and nutritious snack option.

Greek Avocado-Based Snack Recipes

1. Avocado & Feta Greek Toast:

Ingredients:

- 1 ripe avocado

- 2 tablespoons crumbled feta cheese

- 1 teaspoon lemon juice

- Salt and pepper to taste

- 2 slices whole grain bread, toasted

- Cherry tomatoes, sliced (for garnish)

- Fresh basil leaves (for garnish)

Instructions:

1. Mash the ripe avocado in a bowl.

2. Add crumbled feta, lemon juice, salt, and pepper to the mashed avocado. Mix well.

3. Spread the avocado and feta mixture evenly over the toasted whole grain bread slices.

4. Top with sliced cherry tomatoes and fresh basil leaves for a burst of color and flavor.

5. Serve immediately and enjoy your Greek-inspired avocado toast!

2. Greek Avocado & Cucumber Salad:

Ingredients:

- 2 ripe avocados, diced

- 1 cucumber, diced

- 1 cup cherry tomatoes, halved

- 1/4 cup red onion, finely chopped

- 1/3 cup crumbled feta cheese

- 2 tablespoons extra virgin olive oil

- 1 tablespoon red wine vinegar

- 1 teaspoon dried oregano

- Salt and pepper to taste

Instructions:

1. In a large bowl, combine diced avocados, cucumber, cherry tomatoes, red onion, and crumbled feta.

2. In a separate small bowl, whisk together olive oil, red wine vinegar, dried oregano, salt, and pepper to create the dressing.

3. Pour the dressing over the avocado mixture and gently toss until everything is well-coated.

4. Allow the salad to marinate in the refrigerator for about 15 minutes to let the flavors meld.

5. Serve chilled and savor the refreshing Greek Avocado & Cucumber Salad.

3. Avocado & Hummus Stuffed Cucumber Boats:

Ingredients:

- 2 ripe avocados

- 1/2 cup hummus (store-bought or homemade)

- 2 large cucumbers

- Cherry tomatoes, sliced (for garnish)

- Fresh parsley, chopped (for garnish)

- Red pepper flakes (optional, for added spice)

Instructions:

1. Cut the cucumbers in half lengthwise and scoop out the seeds to create cucumber boats.

2. In a bowl, mash the ripe avocados.

3. Mix the mashed avocados with hummus until well combined.

4. Spoon the avocado and hummus mixture into the cucumber boats.

5. Top with sliced cherry tomatoes, chopped fresh parsley, and red pepper flakes if desired.

6. Serve chilled and relish the Avocado & Hummus Stuffed Cucumber Boats as a light and satisfying snack.

These Greek-inspired avocado-based snacks not only provide a delicious burst of flavors but also offer a healthy combination of nutrients. Feel free to customize the recipes to suit your taste preferences, and enjoy these tasty and nutritious treats as part of your balanced diet.

Author Bio

Lucia Diaz Mateo, a distinguished endocrinologist specializing in gestational diabetes and women's health, is the accomplished author behind this comprehensive guide. Holding a Doctorate in Medicine from a renowned institution, Lucia Diaz Mateo,

has dedicated her career to advancing the understanding and management of healthy living.

With a passion for patient-centric care, Lucia Diaz Mateo, combines her extensive clinical experience with a commitment to educating and empowering women. Her research contributions have been widely recognized in leading medical journals, solidifying her position as a respected authority in the field.

www.ingramcontent.com/pod-product-compliance
Lightning Source LLC
Chambersburg PA
CBHW081451250726
48662CB00009B/3038